What YOU Can Do About High Blood Pressure
By Shawn McClendon

Dedication
To my God, to my family, and to my readers.

Table of Contents

Introduction

Several years ago when I was in college, I visited the nearest family health center for a quick check-up. I had felt a small knot in the back of my neck, and while I know now that it was a harmless lymph node, at that time I wasn't sure, so I wanted to get it checked out. Needless to say, I was nervous. Very, very nervous.

Shortly after I was taken to a room to wait for the doctor, the nurse came in to get my vitals. As I sat nervously, the lady wrapped a blood pressure cuff around my arm and took the measurement. "Hmmm…your blood pressure is pretty high," she said as she depressurized the cuff.

Hold up…huh? My blood pressure? High? Nah man, she must've read something wrong because that *can't* be right.

"You said that my blood pressure was high?" I asked for clarification. "Yeah," she said, "but let me take it again to see if it goes down." It did go down *some*, but it was still relatively high. This incident left me somewhat scarred psychologically. I had never, ever had any reason to be concerned about high blood pressure. I was relatively active, young, and thin. There was no high blood pressure in any part of my family to my knowledge. I would later learn that this event made me nervous to get my blood pressure taken at any time, and that nervousness would raise my blood pressure. There is an actual condition for this called White Coat Hypertension (with the white coat being symbolic of the coat doctors wear in the doctor's office).

The same thing happened in another doctor's office a few years later. Almost immediately without asking questions, the doctor said that he could prescribe me a low dose of blood pressure medication, and he made the suggestion as if he expected that I would want or expect a prescription. His suggestion frustrated me because, for one, I've never been very fond of taking medicines unless I really have to, and two, he suggested this without asking me *any* questions about my habits and lifestyle whatsoever. I respectfully declined his offer. These experiences started me on a new personal quest to find out exactly what high blood pressure is and what causes it.

As an African-American, I am sadly aware of how common the disorder is in the African-American community. What I've found is that, while high blood pressure can sometimes be linked to other underlying issues with the body such as kidney problems, this is rare, and for the most part, high blood pressure is characterized as a "lifestyle" disease. The term "lifestyle" disease simply means disease caused by the way a person or a group of people lives, and when I really understood this fact, it truly shocked me. On the other hand, though, it gave me hope.

I have hope because, if high blood pressure can be *caused* by lifestyle, there's a chance that, just maybe, it can be *reversed* by lifestyle as well, once improper lifestyle behaviors are corrected. God built our bodies with an absolutely amazing ability to repair themselves. When we skin our knees, they scab over and new skin is generated. When we break bones, they mend back together. When we exercise and break down our muscles through strength training, they repair and become bigger and stronger. Who's to say that under the right conditions, with the right food, exercise and lifestyle changes, the body can't get its blood pressure back to a normal level? This book is a result of my belief that this can happen and from my desire to help others avoid and prayerfully overcome high blood pressure.

Let me add that this book is not simply based on what I *think* or *hope* for. I researched for accurate information from the National Institutes of Health (NIH), and from studies published in medical journals, as well as from medical websites such as WebMD.com and MayoClinic.com. The information to take charge of high blood pressure is out there, and I have compiled it in this book in an effort to empower you.

Let me leave you with one more important thought that is crucial for you to understand before you read further. Suppose there is a man who is in enormous debt. Now, suppose that this man is a baseball card collector who has recently learned that his collection is worth more than double the amount of debt that he's currently in. Would it be enough for this man to simply be happy that his card collection is worth so much without taking any further action?

Obviously, the answer to that question is a big NO. Unless he likes to be stressed out by having debt, he should waste no time in taking his cards to the right place to cash them in, and then he needs to head to wherever the creditors are to pay off that debt!

My point is, after reading, if you acquire new, helpful knowledge from this book that you believe will help you overcome high blood pressure, please use it. New knowledge won't do you any good otherwise. In Hosea 4:6, God complained through His prophet Hosea about how His people the Israelites were being "destroyed for lack of knowledge." In this case you have the knowledge, so my plea is that we not perish from a failure to use the knowledge we have.

Be blessed,
Shawn McClendon
Back to Basics Health and Wholeness LLC
shawnmcclendon.com

DISCLAIMER: The information in this book is based on my personal opinions, and is not meant to be a substitute for advice from a registered dietitian, nutritionist, doctor or medical professional. You are advised to consult your doctor or physician before incorporating any of the lifestyle changes mentioned in this book.

So What Exactly Is "High Blood Pressure?"

When it comes to dealing with problems of any kind in life, I've increasingly understood that if you really want to deal with a problem, it's not enough to deal with the effects of the problem. You need to understand exactly what the problem is and where it comes from. I realize that just because high blood pressure is common in our country doesn't mean that everybody already knows what it is. With that in mind, let's find out exactly what high blood pressure is.

Regular Ole' Blood Pressure

The term "blood pressure" refers to the force of blood against the walls of blood vessels as the heart pumps it throughout the body. Think of a garden hose. The spigot would essentially represent the heart, and the hose represents your blood vessels. The water flowing through the hose exerts a pressure on the walls of the hose, providing a good representation of blood pressure.

You're probably also familiar with that ratio number associated with blood pressure that your doctor tells you about (i.e. 120/80). That number represents your *systolic* blood pressure over your *diastolic* blood pressure. Ok, so what do those terms mean?

Systolic: Your blood pressure when your heart beats
Diastolic: Your blood pressure in between heart beats

As you see, your systolic blood pressure is higher than your diastolic blood pressure, which is to be expected since in the systolic phase, your heart pumps, and in the diastolic phase, your heart relaxes. Think about that garden hose again. When you turn the spigot on, the hose gets taut. This is somewhat representative of systolic blood pressure. Turning the water off allows the hose to relax, yet water still remains in the hose. This is like diastolic blood pressure.

Another thing to realize about blood pressure is that it is not constant. It changes throughout the day. It drops when you go to sleep, and rises during your waking hours. It goes up when you're excited, stressed, or exercising, and goes down when you take a rest break. Blood pressure is very dynamic.

When It Goes High

Ok, so now that we have a better understanding of what blood pressure is, let's talk *high* blood pressure.

First thing to understand is that there is a such thing as blood pressure being too high. While it is normal for blood pressure to rise with various activities, the rise associated with activities generally is not harmful as it is temporary. However, with high blood pressure (also known as hypertension), the blood pressure remains above 119/79 (below 120/80 is considered normal).

One of the crazy things about high blood pressure is the fact that those who have it are often without symptoms. While some may be alerted to the condition from experiencing dizziness or unusual irritability, many people never know they have it until they get it checked in the doctor's office. Doctors officially diagnose high blood pressure when blood pressure reads high at 2-3 doctor visits.

In other words, you can feel perfectly normal with high blood pressure. This is part of what makes high blood pressure so dangerous. It's elusive.

The Side Effects of Having High Blood Pressure

The other obvious danger of high blood pressure is the damage that it can cause to other parts of the body.

The effects of high blood pressure on blood vessels make me think of rubber bands. Rubber bands can endure a certain amount of stretching without becoming deformed. What happens, though, when you stretch a rubber band too much? It experiences small tears, it loses some of its elasticity, and it can even break.

So it is with blood vessels. They begin to weaken under the continual stress of blood stretching them past their limits, day after day, week after week and year after year. As a result, the organs that blood vessels travel through experience damage. Disorders that can result from having high blood pressure include:

Peripheral Artery Disease
Angina
Heart Attack
Heart Disease
Congestive Heart Failure
Memory Loss
Stroke
Memory Loss
Vision Loss
Kidney Damage

High blood pressure is definitely nothing to take lightly. It does its damage over time, often silently. Once that damage is noticeable, it is often extensive. Even worse, it can result in a catastrophic event such as stroke or heart attack, which can cause permanent bodily damage, if not death.

High Blood Pressure is Way, Way Too Common

In the United States, approximately one out of every three Americans has high blood pressure. That means that if you're in a room with 20 other folks, chances are that at least 7 of you are hypertensive. This is absolutely staggering, especially considering that our American healthcare system is one of the most advanced and the best funded in the world.

And get this. Whereas high blood pressure was generally understood to be an adult disorder, more and more children are being diagnosed. One out of every 25 teenagers has high blood pressure, a trend that experts say is likely due to the rise of obesity in young adults. This is one of the reasons that it has been said in recent years that our generation might be the first generation to have kids with *shorter life spans than their parents*.

To be honest, we all should be outraged by this. To the least, we should be wondering what in the world is going on.

How High Blood Pressure Is Dealt With

When you're diagnosed with high blood pressure, it's best to begin dealing with it as soon as possible to avoid the damage to blood vessels that can result in many of the disorders previously mentioned. Your doctor will definitely want to address it, and will likely recommend and/or prescribe different medications depending on the severity of your condition. Some doctors will recommend lifestyle changes such as salt reduction and exercise.

Speaking of blood pressure medication, I was surprised to learn that there are tons of different kinds that address blood pressure in different ways. In the next chapter, I will detail what I found out about the various medications and how they work. It's important to know about these medicines, especially if you're putting them in your body.

So What's Up With Blood Pressure Medication?

As I stated earlier, I learned that there are many, many different medications used to treat high blood pressure. I initially wondered why and how there could be so many different medicines for one problem, but I found that while all of the medications have the possible end effect of lowering your blood pressure, they do so by suppressing or encouraging different mechanisms in your body. In case you didn't know it, your body is extremely complex, and many bodily processes are involved in regulating your blood pressure. Medications take advantage of this.

The List

Here is the list of medications that I compiled from my research. This list gives the name of each blood pressure medication, as well as what it actually does to possibly lower blood pressure.

Medication Name	What It Does
Thiazide Diuretics (Water Pills)	Reduce blood volume
Beta Blockers	Open blood vessels; cause the heart to beat slower and less hard
Angiotensin-converting Enzyme (ACE) Inhibitors	Block the *formation* of the angiotensin-converting enzyme, which narrows the blood vessels
Angiotensin II Receptor Blockers (ARBs)	Block the *action* of the chemical that narrows the blood vessels
Calcium Channel Blockers	Relax the muscles in the walls of the blood vessels; can also slow the heart rate
Renin Inhibitors	Slow down the production of renin, which is an enzyme in kidneys that can cause blood pressure to rise
Alpha Blockers	Reduce the nerve impulses to blood vessels; Reduce the effect of other

	chemicals that narrow the blood vessels
Alpha-beta Blockers	Reduce the nerve impulses to blood vessels; Slow the heartbeat
Central Acting Agents	Prevent the brain from telling the nervous system to increase heart rate and narrow blood vessels
Vasodilators	Prevent blood vessel muscles from tightening and therefore stop the narrowing of arteries
Aldosterone Antagonists	Block chemical that contributes to salt and fluid retention

As you see, some of these medicines work directly on the blood vessels, some work on the heart, and some work on the nervous system. All produce the same or similar effects by different means. Some medications, like beta blockers, work better when prescribed along with other blood pressure medications. Also, it isn't unusual for a doctor to change a patient's medications depending on how the patient's body initially responds, or if the patient's blood pressure changes and requires an increase or decrease in dosage consequentially.

Important Facts to Understand about the Role of High Blood Pressure Medication

Now, it's really important for us to understand some things about using medication to treat high blood pressure. It simply isn't enough to be diagnosed with it, to get a prescription, and to keep on going. Having high blood pressure in the first place means that something has gone out of whack in the body, and while blood pressure medication can lessen your chances of being hurt by the consequences of high blood pressure, the story does not stop there.

#1: Blood pressure medication does not address the "why" – Yes, you have high blood pressure, and yes, lowering it is good, but *why* do you have blood pressure in the first place? When we experience dysfunction in our bodies, it's never random. There's a good reason for it.

#2: Blood pressure medication does not cure high blood pressure – This builds on my first point. The purpose of high blood pressure medication is simply to lower blood pressure temporarily. That's it. It's important to understand that even if you're taking medication and getting lower blood pressure readings, you still have high blood pressure. That's why you pretty much have to take blood pressure medication *forever*.

#3: Using only blood pressure medication assumes that the body is "broken" – When only medication is used to treat blood pressure, the assumption is that the body no longer has the ability to regulate its own blood pressure. The body is, in essence, "broken" and cannot be repaired. It's similar to putting a patch on a pair of jeans with a hole in the knee, except the patch in this case is the medication.

#4: Using only blood pressure medication allows you to feel dangerously comfortable – Because blood pressure medication lowers blood pressure without addressing the cause of it, it allows us to continue living on as usual. This is dangerous. Why? Because again, when blood pressure is high, it is high for a reason. If, for example, your blood pressure is high due to improper lifestyle habits, blood pressure can give you a false sense of security by causing you to believe that you can live on as usual without changing those habits. This can come back to bite you in the future.

#5: Blood pressure medication has its own list of side effects – I believe that it's always important to know about what you're putting in your body, especially if it can harm you. While medication can keep your blood pressure down, you sign up for the possibility of experiencing the many side effects that can come with taking the medication. To note, anytime you take any medication, there's the possibility that you could experience side effects.

So, what kinds of side effects can occur from taking blood pressure medication? They differ according to the type of medication being taken. For example, cramps can be associated with diuretic medication but they aren't necessarily associated with some of the others. However, I've listed all of the possible side effects together here. They are as follows:

- Harm to pregnant women and fetuses
- Gout
- Leg cramps
- Cold hands and feet
- Insomnia
- Skin rash
- Dizziness
- Headache
- Swollen ankles
- Fever
- Dry mouth
- Diarrhea
- Nightmares
- Allergic reaction
- Impotence
- Weakness
- Fatigue
- Depression
- Dry, hacking cough
- Loss of taste
- Constipation
- Heart palpitations
- Anemia
- Heartburn
- Excessive hair growth

How common are these side effects? I have no statistics, but most sources say that all side effects are generally rare. People likely experience side effects when switching to different blood pressure medications, or when increasing dosage of a medication. So, according to medical sources, side effects are rare; still possible, but rare.

The Sure Way to Avoid All Side Effects

It is only right for me to say that there is treatment for high blood pressure for which there are no detrimental side effects. As a matter of fact, there are *several* things you can do for high blood pressure that will not only help you avoid the effects of high blood pressure and the possible side effects of blood pressure medication, but they can even help you avoid high blood pressure altogether. Some have even reversed their high blood pressure.

One thing that stuck out to me when researching blood pressure medications is that many medical sources agree that blood pressure can be controlled by non-medication means, and that medications should be used when those non-medication means aren't enough.

Here's my thing. I believe that non-medication options are often not emphasized enough for people to really use them. I also believe that there are some people out there, like you, who if given the knowledge to take care of high blood pressure without medication, would jump at the idea and do whatever it takes.

Is that you?

In a couple of chapters, I will talk more on these treatment methods. However, I do want you to understand a few things beforehand:

1. **I am not claiming a definite cure for high blood pressure**. I am not a medical professional and my advice and such should not be taken as if it were from such a professional.

2. **What I have written is not merely based on what I think**. As I said before, I have taken the time to research and compile facts from various sources, several of which are medical websites. See the References page at the end of the book.

3. **Some of these treatment methods I mention later in the book are probably known by your doctor**. As a matter of fact, your doctor may have

even recommended that you do some of these things. However, because doctors practice medicine, their treatment recommendations often involve medicine.

4. **At the end of the day, it'll be up to YOU to take action**. As you'll see, the treatment methods I tell you about can be used by anyone with high blood pressure. However, they also will require a bit of sacrifice on your part. The cool thing is that they don't require the big bucks that medications often require, but on the other hand, they will require you to do something else which can be a challenge, which is…changing your lifestyle.

Before we get into the chapter with the other methods that I'm talking about, I want to encourage you now to have an open mind, and I will be challenging you to give the suggestions a chance. It probably won't be very easy, but then again, nothing that is really worth something comes easily, right?

For now, though, let's first address some of the things that put us at greater risk for having high blood pressure in the first place, AKA risk factors. Once we understand these risk factors, I believe it will be easier for us to understand what kinds of actions to take to truly deal with high blood pressure.

What Puts Me at Greater Risk for Getting High Blood Pressure?

In grade school, I somewhat recall learning the concept of cause and effect. What we were taught was that every effect has a cause. If something happens, that means that another thing *caused* that first thing to happen. If the car doesn't crank and no lights turn on, it's be*cause* the battery is out of juice. The battery is out of juice be*cause* someone left a door open overnight. Someone left the car door open overnight be*cause* they forgot to close it after unloading groceries from the car. See what I mean? Nothing just happens.

And so it is with our physical bodies as it relates to disease. Diseases don't just happen spontaneously. They are caused by something. The causes could be lifestyle-related, environmental, genetic, or even combination of these things.

According to the medical community, there are a number of factors that put people at greater risk for high blood pressure. They're known as "risk factors," and essentially, if people are regularly affected by them, they could contribute to or result in high blood pressure.

Risk factors for high blood pressure are as follows:

- Being African-American
- Being Inactive
- Smoking
- Obesity
- Family History
- Being over 55 years of age
- Using certain medications
- Diabetes
- Excessive Drinking
- High salt consumption

The "Cool" Thing about These Risk Factors

Take a careful look at all of the risk factors and you'll see a common thread between most of them. Do you see it?

If not, let me help you. The common thread that many of the risk factors share is that you have control over them. You decide whether they affect you or not.

Sure, you can't control your race, age and family history, but to some degree you can control every other risk factor. You can control your weight, level of activity, how much you drink, how much salt you consume, and whether or not you smoke.

So if you have high blood pressure but you aren't controlling the factors that you actually can control, you aren't giving your body a fair chance to regulate its own blood pressure.

Isn't it easier now to see how high blood pressure is classified as a <u>lifestyle</u> disease? Lifestyle disease defined is disease caused by how someone lives, and considering how so many of the risk factors are controllable, it makes sense that high blood pressure is among the many diseases caused by lifestyle.

Let me diverge a little bit and talk about a couple of the risk factors that I don't necessarily agree with. I'll explain why.

About African-American Race Being a Risk Factor

I must say that while most of the risk factors make sense to me in regards to contributing to high blood pressure, one in particular doesn't make any sense at all to me. That risk factor is being African-American.

Yes, we as African-Americans are disproportionately affected by high blood pressure, as we are with many other lifestyle diseases. However, I disagree that it simply has to do with being black. It doesn't make sense to me that being black can contribute to high blood pressure in the same way that smoking or being inactive can. To say that one race of people is more prone to high blood pressure than others doesn't quite add up to me.

I believe that African-Americans are more often affected by high blood pressure, not because of our race, but because of two main things:

1. A greater proportion of African-Americans are unable to afford quality, healthy foods, and therefore purchase and eat larger amounts of processed, disease promoting foods

2. Lower income makes African-Americans more likely to experience more of the risk factors that contribute to high blood pressure.

Needless to say, I do not agree that simply being African-Americans puts us at a greater risk.

About Family History Being a Risk Factor

I also believe that saying that family history is a risk factor can at least be misleading. While it is true that family history can sometimes influence our susceptibility to certain diseases, family history is by no means a definite sign that we'll contract a disease. Scientists have said that our lifestyles can determine whether or not certain genes express themselves or not, meaning that the way that you live still has a greater bearing on whether or not you get sick with something.

Think about this as well. Is it possible that part of what causes lifestyle diseases like high blood pressure, diabetes and obesity to run in families is learned behavior? If a child grows up in a family where both parents are dealing with high blood pressure as a result of unhealthy habits, chances are that the child isn't going to live differently. The child is going to adopt the same unhealthy habits as his or her parents, which I think we can agree will make the child much more likely to suffer from high blood pressure as well.

I wonder if "family history" should be "family habits" instead. What do you think?

I'm Ready to Know What I Can Do

Ok, don't worry. We're about to get into what everyone wants to know, which is, "What can I actually do myself about high blood pressure?" What I found, and what you will find, is that there is plenty that you can do to treat your own high blood pressure, and it's only right for you to give yourself a full chance to let your body regulate itself by giving your body what it's always needed before you sign up for taking blood pressure medication for the rest of your life. Let's go.

Strategies for Dealing with Your Own Blood Pressure

Ok, let me preface this chapter by saying this. There are several, and I mean *several*, things you can do on your own that can possibly lower your blood pressure. You may already know about some of these methods, and there may be some you never heard about. Your doctor may know of some too, and may have even told you about them already.

Let me ask you a question. When you were diagnosed with high blood pressure (if you have been diagnosed), did you try to do everything you could in your own strength to lower it before resorting to medication? I'm not talking about lowering your sodium for a couple of days and then saying that it doesn't work. I'm talking about putting in a concerted, all-in effort to do the right things for your body to give it a chance to right itself.

My next question is, did your doctor tell you about non-medication actions you could take before prescribing medicine to you? Granted, I believe that some of them do. Many doctors sit with their patients and explain how things like lowering sodium, exercising, and following the DASH diet will help.

On the other hand, I know that there are other doctors out there who won't say anything about what you can do apart from medicine. As I said in the Introduction, when I had a higher-than-normal blood pressure reading at the doctor's office, he immediately suggested that he could prescribe me a low dose of high blood pressure medication to see how I would respond. He said absolutely nothing about things like exercise, sodium intake and relaxation, to name a few. Only after I asked him if I could just change some lifestyle habits did he respond, "oh, you can do that too."

Look, to be honest, whether your doctor is a great doctor or not, he or she doesn't own your body. It's the truth. One of the sayings I've adopted is "My Doctor Isn't Responsible for My Health…I AM." It's my body, given to **me** by God, so I make the final decisions about what I do with it…not my doctor. This is why it is so important that we take responsible measures to keep ourselves healthy. We're the ones who are personally responsible.

The List

Before we go into detail, I want to list out eight things that you can focus on changing if your blood pressure is high. All of these are lifestyle changes that anyone can make, and they are as follows:

1. Exercise
2. Lose Excess Body Fat
3. Eat Less Sodium
4. Eat More Potassium
5. Eat Less Meat
6. Drink More Water
7. Practice Slow, Deep Breathing
8. Get Enough Sleep

9. Get Flexible

Pretty simple, isn't it? I wouldn't be surprised if it seems almost too simple. Think about it, though. At the end of the day, the focus with each of these methods is on getting your body back where it needs to be by giving it what it's always needed. Like any machine, our bodies are always in need of various kinds of fuel and maintenance, without which they will malfunction. While medicine has its place, simply using medicine doesn't acknowledge this fact. Medicine doesn't give your body what it's always needed. It only lowers your blood pressure.

Let's explore each of these eight methods in detail to see why they can help you lower your blood pressure.

Exercise

You probably already knew that exercise was good for lowering blood pressure. Exercise demands greater usage of the heart and lungs, and while blood pressure increases during such activity, regular exercise has the desirable effect of lowering your blood pressure over time.

Regular exercise increases the efficiency of your heart and your lungs and results in a greater level of maximal oxygen consumption, which is the point at which your consumption of oxygen peaks when you're doing more work. In other words, your body has the capacity to take in more oxygen with less effort. This is important because your blood is responsible for transporting oxygen around your body, and if your body can transport more oxygen around with less blood, your body is definitely becoming more efficient. Exercise also has an indirect effect on lowering your blood pressure by decreasing your body fat, which I talk about in the next section.

Exercising regularly has been shown to especially lower the blood pressure of individuals with moderate high blood pressure. This is good news for you. And get this: If you're currently sedentary, you can receive the benefit of lower blood pressure with a very small amount of exercise.

A study published in the Journal of Human Hypertension guided several sedentary individuals through a very minimal amount of exercise. The test subjects were required to exercise only 30-60 minutes per week, and they experienced what was termed as "clinically significant" decreases in their blood pressure. In other words, they were exercising only 5-10 minutes a day, 6 days per week, and experiencing drops in their blood pressure. That's phenomenal.

While you should aim for a minimum of 150 minutes of aerobic exercise per week, or 30 minutes 5 days per week, the most important thing to remember is that if you aren't already exercising and you have high blood pressure, you just need to get started. Start with just 5 minutes a day, and do it consistently. It helps!

Lose Excess Body Fat

In men, the percentage of body fat considered essential is 2-5%. That percentage is 10-13% for women. The average person doesn't need to worry about getting too close to these body fat percentages unless you desire to be ripped with a 6-pack, but on the other hand, you must understand that having too much body fat increases the amount of strain on the heart, causing the heart to have to pump harder to deliver blood and oxygen to the rest of the body. Excess body fat is the culprit in the case of obesity, which is defined as over 25% body fat in men, and over 32% body fat in women.

Lowering your body fat lessens the load on your heart and allows it to more efficiently supply your body with oxygen, which means less work for your heart, and possibly lower blood pressure. You can lower your body fat by eating a diet based on lots of vegetables and fruits and by exercising, among other things. When I say "based on lots of vegetables and fruits", I mean that the foundation of your diet should be plant foods.

Eat Less Sodium

The admonition to "watch your salt" is something that all people with high blood pressure are likely very familiar with. Hopefully, you have already paid attention to this because consuming too much salt can definitely be detrimental to your blood pressure.

Here's why. Your kidneys, which filter the fluid in your body to get rid of waste, require a delicate balance of sodium and potassium. Having that right balance of these two elements allows your kidneys to efficiently pull water from the bloodstream. Getting extra water out of the bloodstream is important for blood pressure, because too much water in the blood means a higher blood volume and more pressure on the blood vessel walls...in other words, higher blood pressure. That's why doctors prescribe diuretics which pull extra water out of the body.

As stated before, however, diuretics don't necessarily address the real issue when it comes to the body retaining water. When we consume too much sodium, we upset the balance of sodium and potassium in our kidneys, preventing them from pulling water out of the blood like they should. As expected, the best way to address this is by consuming less salt.

It is very, very common for individuals to consume too much salt. Sodium naturally occurs in many foods, so it's wise to be sparing when it comes to adding more sodium in the form of salt. If you regularly use the salt shaker at the dinner table, it's likely that you're eating too much sodium. If you consume a lot of processed, packaged foods, especially like frozen dinners and processed meat, you could definitely be getting more sodium than you need to. Focusing on consuming fresher foods and seasoning them with different herbs and spices (like garlic powder) will help you to diversify your palate and reduce your sodium without sacrificing taste. So don't be scared to go experiment with spices. Some of my favorite foods are the different ethnic foods that rely on various spices instead of salt and taste great.

You can also get that balance of sodium and potassium in your kidneys where it needs to be by consuming more potassium, which I'll talk about next.

Eat More Potassium

As stated before, the kidneys require an appropriate balance of sodium and potassium to pull water from the blood effectively. When we add salt to our meals, it becomes easy to upset that balance. Therefore, another way to restore the balance and therefore potentially lower blood pressure is to increase the amount of potassium in your diet.

Now, obviously we don't sprinkle potassium onto our food like we do with sodium (in the form of salt). If we could, however, it probably wouldn't be wise to do so. The reason is because it is very easy to overdo it with potassium. Doctors advise against taking it in supplemental form. So how in the world do we increase potassium safely?

It's simple. Eat your vegetables and fruits.

Plant foods naturally contain good amounts of potassium. It's always better to get all of your nutrients, including potassium, in natural form because the nutrients are better assimilated and in the appropriate amounts. In other words, God knew what he was doing when he made plants for our consumption.

The potassium in plant foods isn't the only reason we should consume more of them. Plant-based diets that especially include lots of leafy greens and "watery" vegetables like tomatoes, cucumbers and squash make it easy to lose weight. They are naturally low in calories and high in nutrients. You can eat lots of them until you're full and never have to worry about eating too many calories. When you eat fewer calories, you lose extra fat, and less fat means lower blood pressure.

So if you're not abiding by grandma's age old admonition to "eat your vegetables," it is high time to do so. It could help lower your blood pressure.

Eat Less Meat

Contrary to cultural norms, we don't need nearly as much meat as we normally eat in the U.S. We're accustomed to having sausage or bacon for breakfast, maybe some deli meat on a sandwich for lunch, and a steak or a chicken breast for dinner, but consider this. Certain animals like dogs and cats are much better suited for meat-based diets, as evidenced by their mouthfuls of canine teeth. We, on the other hand, contain only four canine teeth which are dull when compared to those of animals. We contain many more molars, which are teeth designed for grinding…guess what? Plant foods.

To add, The China Study, which was conducted by T. Colin Campbell, suggests that high consumption of animal protein greatly increases cholesterol levels in the blood and leads to buildup of plaques in the blood vessels, otherwise known as atherosclerosis. The atherosclerosis buildup narrows the blood vessels and consequentially raises the blood pressure. It also opens the door to more dangerous diseases and disorders like heart disease and heart attack.

The study suggested further that eating a plant-based diet does well with lowering cholesterol levels in the body, and can possibly even reduce the plaques in blood vessels, which can lower the blood pressure, and the study even suggested that a plant-based diet can reverse heart disease. Needless to say, The China Study is a good read if you don't mind reading detailed studies.

Eat meat occasionally while making plant protein sources like beans and nuts your main go-to sources of protein. Experiment with making at least one day a meatless day. Better yet, try going on a fast from meat for a few days. You might be surprised how many different things you can do with vegetables, and you might even find yourself not really missing meat. Hey, don't laugh!

Drink More Water

We know that water pills lower blood pressure by helping to pull water out of the body and therefore lowering blood volume, but another common way of pulling water out of the body is by drinking more water.

It seems counterintuitive, but it's true. Oftentimes, our bodies retain water because they just aren't getting enough of it. It's essentially a survival mechanism. It kinda makes me think about how camels hold water in the humps in their backs. Hey, I'm not calling you a camel.

Anyhow, when we supply our bodies with plenty of water, they no longer need to hold on to it and very readily purge it. Those who have attempted to increase their water intake know what I'm talking about. When you first increase your water intake, you'll have to go to the restroom seemingly all of the time, but eventually your body gets accustomed to it.

The cool thing about it is that when you're getting in enough water, not only are you potentially lowering your blood pressure, but you're also keeping your body fully hydrated. Diuretic medications do pull extra water out of your body, but they do not help keep you hydrated..

The age old recommendation is to drink 8-10 8 oz glasses of the best quality of water you can find every day.

Practice Slow, Deep Breathing

Do this little experiment. Place one hand on your chest and another on your belly. As you breathe, take note of which hand moves the most. Is it the hand on your chest? If so, you're more of a chest breather, which means that you're not breathing deep enough. If the hand on your stomach moves more, that means that you are expanding your diaphragm as you should to take good, deep breaths.

Here's another experiment. As you go throughout your workday, pay attention to how you're breathing. Do you ever notice yourself holding your breath? You might be surprised. For many people, it's common to hold their breath several times a day, especially in stressful, fast-paced work environments.

Our stressful lives often cause us to forget how to breathe correctly. Instead of taking slower "belly" breaths that fully expand our diaphragms, we become accustomed to taking quick, shallow breaths, and we even unconsciously hold our breath at times. All of this can possibly have a negative effect on your blood pressure.

Have you ever noticed how when you inhale, your pulse generally gets faster and stronger, and when you exhale, your pulse slows and becomes more gentle? This is because inhalation and exhalation are controlled by two different aspects of your nervous system, which are your Sympathetic Nervous System and your Parasympathetic Nervous System, respectively. The Sympathetic Nervous System is responsible for your "fight or flight" response to dangerous or stressful situations. When you live a life filled with stress, that fight or flight response is activated often, causing increases in pulse rate and blood pressure. Over time, your body becomes more sensitive to this response, making it easier for you to respond in this manner.

The Parasympathetic Nervous System is responsible for your relaxation response. Anytime you exhale, you activate this relaxation response, which is why slow, deep breathing exercises are important. These kinds of exercises allow you to tone a nerve responsible for the relaxation response, called the Vagus nerve. You essentially train that nerve so that your body returns to a more constant, relaxed state.

Breathing exercises that will help in this manner will usually have an exhalation phase that is twice as long as the inhalation phase. The 4-7-8 Breathing Exercise from Dr. Weil is a good example, allowing for 4 seconds of inhalation, 7 seconds to hold the breath, and 8 seconds for exhalation. If done correctly, you will immediately feel relaxed, and over time your blood pressure can decrease.

A study in the Journal of Human Hypertension guided patients through musically-guided deep breathing exercises for 8 weeks at 10 minutes per day. Over half of the participants had a 7.5 mm/4.0mm drop in their blood pressures after the study, leading the conductors of the study to conclude that deep breathing is an "effective non-pharmacological treatment for high blood pressure.

In other words, practicing deep breathing is an effective way to treat your blood pressure without drugs.

You might be interested in looking into a device called Resperate. Apparently, it is a device that uses music to guide your breaths in such a way to show you how to breathe deeply. It has been shown to help lower blood pressure, and the cool thing about it is that you don't need a prescription for it. Look it up!

Get Enough Sleep

Sleep is not just important to get so that you're not tired. It's one of the most crucial, if not the most crucial, things you can do for your health, and could possibly have an effect on your blood pressure.

When you sleep, your body enters a highly important stage of repair. Your body is repairing cells as well as regulating and releasing various hormones important for rejuvenating the body. When you skip sleep, you short circuit this whole process, and it's actually quite stressful for your body.

This stress causes the release of cortisol, often referred to as the "stress hormone." Cortisol is meant to help our bodies react to stressful, "fight or flight" situations, but when we make a practice of skipping sleep, cortisol is constantly being released into our bodies, which weren't made to always have cortisol floating around. This makes for an almost constant level of stress.

As far as stress and blood pressure are concerned, stress temporarily elevates the blood pressure. Over time, however, excessive exposure to stress hormones does harm to our bodies by keeping our blood pressure elevated more than it should be. Excessive cortisol levels also can do harm to cognition and the cardiovascular system, and can cause fat accumulation which is yet another contributor to high blood pressure.

More missed sleep means more exposure to stress hormones, and this also means more constantly elevated blood pressure levels. If you're taking blood pressure medicine but not giving yourself something as practical as a good night's sleep, I encourage you to give yourself a chance by getting your rest. Most people should be getting somewhere between seven and nine hours of sleep each night, so make that your goal. Make it a goal as well to not have to use an alarm clock. Apparently, if you have to use one, it probably means you're not getting enough sleep.

I believe that it's no coincidence that sleep disorders like sleep apnea are often associated with high blood pressure. Sleep is extremely important, so get enough of it if you aren't already.

Get Flexible

Have you tried touching your toes lately?

If you are currently unable to touch your toes while doing a sit-and-reach stretch – where you sit down with your legs straight in front of you while reaching forward to touch your feet – that could be contributing to higher blood pressure.

Consider this: Your muscles are filled with blood vessels. If those muscles are stiff, that means that the blood vessels within them are stiff as well, and therefore, the blood flow within them is restricted.

The flexibility of your trunk (midsection) is key. If you are unable to bend your trunk enough to touch your toes, according to a study in the *SpringerPlus* journal, that is a good indicator that major arteries in your body are inflexible and stiff. Your leg muscles, the largest muscles in your body, can also constrict blood vessels and raise blood pressure, which is important in particular because your legs are furthest away from your heart, and therefore, the vessels require significant flexibility to move the blood through.

In the study, participants who engaged in four weeks of stretching, which included the sit-and-reach test, significantly reduced their arterial stiffness. Another study in the *Journal of Physical Activity and Health* showed that stretching may be more effective for lowering blood pressure than walking.

That said, stretch! Making full-body stretching part of your regular routine is the key to seeing any results. Stretching is already a very valuable practice since it helps you to maintain your mobility as you age, so the possibility of consistent stretching lowering your blood pressure is a nice added benefit.

A Cool Thing About These Self-Treatment Methods

While researching for this chapter, I noticed something very interesting with the various lifestyle changes I just mentioned.

What I'm talking about is the fact that many of these lifestyle changes work in more than one way to possibly help you lower your blood pressure naturally…

- Exercising can help lower the blood pressure by **conditioning the heart and lungs**, and by **getting rid of body fat**
- Consuming more potassium by eating a plant-based diet can help lower the blood pressure by **restoring the sodium/potassium balance in your kidneys**, which helps prevent water retention, and by **lowering your body fat** due to less calorie consumption
- Eating less meat can help lower the blood pressure by **reducing plaque buildup in the arteries**, allowing the blood to flow more freely, and by **making room for more potassium (plant food) consumption**, which helps in the ways stated in the previous bullet point
- Drinking more water can help lower the blood pressure by **reducing water retention**, and by **lowering your body fat due to less calorie consumption** (since water helps you feel full)
- Getting enough sleep can help lower the blood pressure by **reducing the level of stress your**

body is under. This decreases your cortisol levels, and less cortisol means **less body fat accumulation**, which can help lower your blood pressure as well.

- Stretching lowers your blood pressure by **reducing arterial stiffness in the trunk and legs**, and it also can reduce stress indirectly by **loosening stiff muscles and leading you to breathe deeply**

Isn't it wonderful how so many of these work together?

Here's the thing. None of the strategies that I've told you about are really profound or groundbreaking, which is precisely what makes them so important to consider if you truly want to get control of your blood pressure. All of these are things that you and I should already be doing.

In the next and final chapter, we're going to discuss the most important thing in this book, which is how to implement what we've just learned. The greatest knowledge in the world is pretty much worthless if it is never used. In the same manner, if you store all of the knowledge you've learned from this book and never use it, it will be of no use to you.

A Plan to Implement Blood Pressure Control Strategies

In the previous chapter, we outlined eight easy-to-implement strategies that you can take that can lower your blood pressure. Let us now talk about how to implement these strategies.

Let's Get Real

Ok, so we're all adults here. We all know by now that zeal by itself is almost never enough to make us change our behaviors.

When I was an undergraduate in college, before the start of each semester, I always had the desire to begin studying well before school began again, and to continue superb study habits throughout the whole semester to hopefully guarantee that I would make an 'A' in each class.

Ha!

What did I do instead? Every time, I overestimated how much time I had before school started, and I procrastinated as a result. By the time school would begin, I had usually only studied about a week or so to the most, and because my classes were hard, I found myself playing catch-up over and over again. It's really pretty sad.

What I'm saying is, I know how it is to really want to do something, to say you're going to do something, and to not do it. I also know how it is to repeat that cycle over and over again. I don't want you to fall into the same trap.

Is It Important?

We need to ask ourselves this question when we endeavor to replace bad habits with new ones: Is it important that I adopt this new behavior? Is it really important? And by important, I mean, is it absolutely crucial that you adopt these new habits for your wellbeing?

Since we're talking about blood pressure in this book, ask yourself this question...

Is it really important that I make changes in my life that can possibly lower my blood pressure?

Well, let's think about it. We discussed earlier how high blood pressure can lead to a number of life-threatening diseases and conditions, including heart attack and stroke. Let's go further.

Now, having high blood pressure that contributes to other life-threatening diseases wouldn't matter if our lives were insignificant, but see, that's the thing. Your life IS significant. Because you are the only somebody like you in this entire world, you have something different to offer than anybody else can. To me, that means you are far too significant to have your life shortened by a treatable and potentially reversible disorder like high blood pressure.

So yes, I would say that it is definitely important that you, yes **you**, make whatever changes that you need to make to your lifestyle to lower your blood pressure.

Your Game Plan

If you're a subscriber to my blog
(shawnmcclendon.com), read my first book
(13 Things to Stop Believing to Become
Healthy and Lose Weight), or done one of my
online workout programs, you know by now
that I'm not the kind of guy who
recommends "cold turkey" changes.

I do believe that if you make your mind up,
you can implement all eight lifestyle changes
I've discussed in the previous chapter at the
same. People do it all the time.

However, the truth is that many of us, myself
included, become overwhelmed by having to
make too many changes at once, and we
might start out okay, but we are most likely
to crash and burn.

Because of that, I've set up a gradual game plan for you to follow to implement all eight changes. The duration of this plan is four weeks, which will have you making two changes each week. These changes will add up cumulatively until you've implemented all changes by the end of Week 4.

Now, it's going to be important that you monitor your blood pressure throughout these four weeks. This way, you will be able to see whether or not these changes are beginning to naturally lower your blood pressure.

Finally, and most importantly, you should tell your doctor about everything that you're doing. My advice is not to be taken as advice from a doctor or medical professional. Your doctor should be notified about any changes you make. On top of that, if your blood pressure goes down due to you making changes in your lifestyle, your doctor will need to know so that he/she can reduce, and perhaps eventually eliminate, your blood pressure medication. This is really important.

On to the plan.

Week 1: Sleep and Deep Breathing

- Adjust your bed time so that you are getting no less than 7.5 hours in the bed every single night

    o Bed Time:_____ Rise Time:_____

- Take two 5 minute breaks every day (e.g. mid-morning at work, after work, prayer time, etc.) to do the following:

    o Find a quiet, dark place if possible

    o Sit upright in a chair or on the floor

    o Inhale through your nose for 4 seconds, while placing your hand on your abdomen to

ensure you're breathing from
your belly

- ○ Hold the breath briefly
- ○ Release the breath through lips
  (in 'o' shape) over 8 seconds
- ○ Relax for a moment, then begin
  again with another inhale.
  Repeat until your 5 minutes
  have elapsed

**None of this should be
uncomfortable**

Week 2: More Water, Less Sodium

- Start and end your day with two tall
  glasses of the best water you can find

- Refrain from using salt shakers at the table

- Reduce your intake of restaurant food/fast food/frozen dinners to no more than 2-3 meals for the whole week so that you can regulate your sodium by cooking your own food

-----

Week 3: More Potassium, Less Meat

- Make every Monday a Meatless Monday (check out MeatlessMonday.com for ideas)

- Make no less than half of your plate at every meal consist of plant foods

- For breakfast, you can consume a couple of pieces of fruit or a fresh fruit bowl with sliced bananas, grapes, pineapple, strawberries, etc. (no canned fruits)
- For lunch and dinner, choose leafy and/or "watery" vegetables for half of your plate. Choices include onions, peppers, spinach, collards, cabbage, turnip greens, broccoli, cauliflower, asparagus, tomatoes, squash, okra

- Make big pots of brown rice (not instant) and dried beans of your choice (pinto, black, red kidney, etc.), and eat this for your meat for lunch and/or dinner until it runs out. After that runs out, you can eat meat. Your wallet or pocketbook is going to thank you for this one ;)

Week 4: Exercise and Reduce Fat

- Start walking for 5 minutes every single day
    - Your Daily Walk

        Time:_____ AM/PM

- Increase your walk time by one minute every week, at least until you reach 30 minutes each day. I challenge you to aim for one hour each day...you can split it into different times each day

- Add nightly stretching to your routine. Include sit-and-reach, standing hamstring stretch, calf stretch, arm across the chest, doorway chest stretch, and gentle neck stretches to the front, back and sides

- Replace all sweet drinks (sweet tea, soda, flavored water, juices, etc.) with water

- Eat grains (brown rice, whole grain breads and pastas, etc.) no more than once a day. After that, replace them with leafy and/or watery vegetables

Conclusion

Dear reader, my most sincere desire is that this booklet has not only informed you about the many ways you can change your lifestyle to affect your blood pressure in a good way, but also, that it has empowered you to take action right now to make a healthier life a reality for you.

Although I am a personal trainer, I didn't write this book as a personal trainer. Rather, I wrote this book as a regular person who has noticed information out there about possibly overcoming high blood pressure that I feel is not emphasized enough. Yes, we're told about how important it is that we get high blood pressure treated, and that's correct. However, more than anything we are encouraged to take medicine for high blood pressure. Because high blood pressure is classified as a lifestyle disease, I feel that it is important first that we are encouraged to make every effort to correct our lifestyles, and *then* see how much we really need medication after that. Doesn't that make sense?

Why spend money on medication if it ends up that we really don't have to spend that money?

Why expose ourselves to the side effects of medication if it turns out that we really don't need the medicine?

Why allow ourselves to keep on living lives that promote disease if we can make a few sacrifices that promote quality and quantity of life? These are the kinds of questions I encourage you to think about here at the conclusion of this book.

I really appreciate your investment in this book and hope you enjoyed it. However, my goal is not simply to provide you with an enjoyable book. Please, take whatever you've learned in this book and put it to use. Give your body a chance by giving it what it's always needed – rest, water, lots of plant foods, less meat, less stress, and so on – and see if your body responds favorably.

A coworker and friend of mine who has dealt with high blood pressure told me about how he began to practice deep breathing just before he would take his blood pressure at one of the machines commonly seen in stores, gyms and workplaces. Whenever he did that, his blood pressure would drop significantly from that alone. He still is in the process of changing some other habits in his life that might contribute, but deep breathing alone has had a significant impact.

Give it a chance. I challenge you to employ all of the strategies mentioned in this book and see what happens. And if you are helped, I ask that you would tell somebody else with high blood pressure about the book so that they can be helped as well.

I invite you to follow me by subscribing to my e-mail list at https://shawnmcclendon/subscribe. You will receive my periodic posts on health and fitness, wholeness, and other related topics that I'm interested in.

You can also follow me on Instagram at @shawnb2bfitness and on Facebook at @shawnb2b.

If this plan helps you, I'd love to hear about it from you. Please consider leaving an honest review of this book on Amazon.com. I would greatly appreciate it.

God bless you.

References

"What is High Blood Pressure?" *National Heart, Lung and Blood Institute* . National Heart, Lung and Blood Institute, 2 August 2012. Web. 15 August 2015.

"Why Blood Pressure Matters." *American Heart Association.* American Heart Association, 13 August 2014. Web. 15 August 2015.

"Understanding High Blood Pressure -- the Basics." *WebMD.* WebMD, 28 February 2015. Web. 15 August 2015.

"Salt and blood pressure: Cutting down on the white stuff could save your life." *Blood Pressure UK.* Blood Pressure UK. Web. 15 August 2015.

"The Physiology of Stress: Cortisol and the Hypothalamic-Pituitary-Adrenal Axis." Dartmouth Undergraduate Journal of Science, 3 February 2011. Web. 15 August 2015.

Grossman, E, Grossman, A, Schein, MH, Zimlichman, R and B Gavish. "Breathing-control lowers blood pressure." *Journal of Human Hypertension* 15 (2001): 263–269. Print.

"High blood pressure (hypertension): Treatments and drugs." *Mayo Clinic.* Mayo Clinic, 7 July 2015. Web. 15 August 2015.

"How much exercise is required to reduce blood pressure in essential hypertensives: a dose-response study." *American Journal of Hypertension* (2001). Web. 15 August 2015.

"Breathing: Three Exercises." *DrWeil.com.* DrWeil.com. Web. 15 August 2015.

Hanson, Rick PhD. "Relaxed and Contented: Activating the Parasympathetic Wing of Your Nervous System." 2007.

"Hosea 4." *Bible Gateway.* Bible Gateway. Web. 18 August 2015.

Bryant, Cedric X. PhD and Green, Daniel J. *ACE'S Essentials of Exercise Science for Fitness Professionals.* American Council on Exercise, 2012. Print.

"High Blood Pressure (Hypertension)." *KidsHealth*. The Nemours Foundation. Web. 8 September 2015.

"Side Effects of High Blood Pressure Medications." *WebMD*. WebMD, 12 April 2015. Web. 10 September 2015.

Nishiwaki M, Yonemura H, Kurobe K, Matsumoto N. Four weeks of regular static stretching reduces arterial stiffness in middle-aged men. Springerplus. 2015 Sep 25;4:555. doi: 10.1186/s40064-015-1337-4. PMID: 26435901; PMCID: PMC4583555.

Ko, J., Deprez, D., Shaw, K., Alcorn, J., Hadjistavropoulos, T., Tomczak, C., Foulds, H., & Chilibeck, P. D. (2021). Stretching is Superior to Brisk Walking for Reducing Blood Pressure in People With High–Normal Blood Pressure or Stage I Hypertension, JOURNAL OF PHYSICAL ACTIVITY AND HEALTH, 18(1), 21-28. Retrieved Jul 15, 2022, from https://journals.humankinetics.com/view/journals/jpah/18/1/article-p21.xml

About the Author

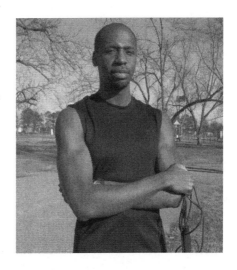

Shawn McClendon is an ACE Certified Personal Trainer, owner of shawnmcclendon.com, a fitness writer for *Macon Magazine* and a former columnist for *The Macon Telegraph*. He is also the author of several books, including *13 Things to Stop Believing to Become Healthy and Lose Weight*.

Employed by day as an Electronics Engineer, Shawn spends time outside of his day job instructing and educating others on how to live healthier lives out of a strong desire to see others live better. He sees this as a ministry through which to spread God's love to others in need. In addition to writing and conducting small group personal training sessions, he also speaks to groups on health and fitness related topics.

To have Shawn to speak to your group in person or virtually on health/fitness topics including preventing lifestyle-caused diseases and Physical Fitness, e-mail shawn@shawnmcclendon.com.

He lives in Georgia with his wife and daughters.

Printed in Great Britain
by Amazon

36306412R00046